THE HABIT REVOLUTION

A Women's Guide to Evolving Health, Habits, and Hormones, from First Period to Post Menopause

Sarah Boyd

Lucky Book Publishing

MY GIFT TO YOU

I am so glad you're here!

As my Gift to you, get FREE Access to the Audiobook of The Habit Revolution and other bonus content by scanning the QR Code below or visiting sarahboyd.ca

MY DREAM

My dream is to take the mystery out of health and put the power back in your hands. Too many people feel stuck in the cycle of quick fixes, fad diets, and workouts that burn you out instead of build you up. I want to change that by teaching the basics -the big three that truly matter: how you move, how you fuel, and how you recover.

I dream of a world where health literacy is as common as learning to read. Where women know exactly how to move their bodies to feel strong and capable at every age. Where food isn't a source of stress, but fuel that powers you through busy days and celebrations alike. Where sleep isn't seen as optional, but respected as one of the most powerful training tools you have.

I dream of women who understand that fitness doesn't have to mean hours in the gym, that nutrition doesn't mean cutting out entire food groups, and that recovery isn't laziness, it's progress. Health doesn't come from extremes; it comes from stacking small, smart choices until they become second nature. Motion is lotion. Food is fuel. Sleep is training.

Most of all, I dream of women who trust themselves; who know that walking counts, lifting counts, laughter counts, and yes even rest days count! Women who feel confident passing that knowledge on to their daughters, sisters, and friends. My dream is to create ripples of health literacy that spread wider than any workout plan ever could.

Yours in health and wellness,

Sarah

INTRODUCTION

Why We Need a Habit Revolution for Women

We're living in an exciting time for women's health. After decades of being underrepresented in research, more studies are now being done *by* and *for* women than ever before. Scientists, coaches, and clinicians are uncovering how female physiology, hormones, and metabolism actually work; and it's transforming how we think about training, nutrition, recovery, and habit formation.

This new wave of research is showing what many women have always sensed: we aren't just smaller versions of men. Our hormone cycles influence everything from our energy and sleep to how we respond to exercise and stress. Understanding these differences isn't about limitation, it's about optimization and efficiency. It means women can finally build routines and habits that align with our natural rhythms instead of fighting against them to fit into a mold that doesn't feel right.

Dr. Stacy Sims coined the term "shrink it and pink it" to describe the old approach to women's health: when programs and products were simply scaled down and rebranded instead of reimagined. Thankfully, that era is ending. Today, experts like Sims and countless others are leading a new wave of female-focused science that celebrates women's physiology and gives us the tools to train, eat, and live in sync with it.

It's no wonder so many women have felt frustrated, they're doing everything "right" yet still feeling stuck, tired, or out of sync. Your body isn't working against you; it's simply asking for a different kind of support. When your approach matches how your body actually works, everything changes. Energy returns. Progress feels natural. And taking care of yourself becomes something that flows, not something you have to force.

That's why this book exists. *The Habit Revolution* tosses out the one-size-fits-all wellness playbook and helps you create your own playbook that actually fits YOU. It's about learning to listen when your body is whispering at you, instead of waiting until it's screaming. It's about building habits that flow with your biology instead of against it. Whether you're just starting out, navigating a new phase of life, or trying to figure out why your usual strategies aren't working anymore, you're in the right place.

How this Book Works: Read what Applies to you Now and What's Coming Later

This book is divided into four parts, and you don't have to read it in order (but you can if you would like!) . It's meant to be more of a choose-your-own-adventure kind of guide. Dip in where it makes sense for you right now, and come back to the rest when the time comes.

- **Part I** lays the groundwork: how women's bodies and hormones actually work, why that matters for habit change, and what the core pillars of wellness look like when they're tailored to you.

- **Parts II, III, and IV** are based on the major stages of a woman's life: adolescence, the reproductive years, and the menopause transition. Start with the section that reflects where you're at today, or get a head start on what's coming next.

You will find practical tips, real-life stories, and habit strategies you can use: no overhauls, no shame, no nonsense. Just tools to help you feel more at home in your body and more confident in your choices.

This isn't about hustling harder. It's about syncing up with your body, your cycle, and your season of life so you can build habits that *actually* stick.

Ready?

Let's start the revolution.

CONTENTS

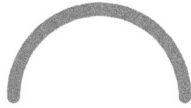

PART I
FOUNDATIONS OF
FEMALE HABIT BUILDING

CHAPTER 1
THE FEMALE BODY EXPLAINED

If you've ever thought, *"Why didn't I learn this in school*, you're not alone. Our education about the female body often skips the most important stuff: how our biology impacts energy, performance, mood, and habits. These things aren't random, they're rhythmic, and once you understand the patterns, you can unlock the code.

Meet the Female Sex Hormones

Before we dive into the phases of your cycle, let's talk about the hormones that run the show. The primary female sex hormones: **estrogen**, **progesterone**, and **testosterone** are powerful chemical messengers that influence everything from your metabolism to your mood. They don't just affect your reproductive system; they impact your brain, your muscles, your bones, your sleep, your stress response, and even your motivation.

Estrogen is often thought of as the star of

the show. It rises in the first half of your cycle and plays a huge role in making you feel more energetic, social, and cognitively sharp. It also helps with muscle building, insulin sensitivity, and mood regulation.

Progesterone takes the lead in the second half of your cycle. It's known for its calming, grounding effect, but it can cause fatigue, bloating, or brain fog if it's out of balance. Progesterone prepares your body for rest and recovery and is a key player in managing inflammation and nervous system regulation.

Testosterone is generally thought of as a "male" hormone, but it plays an important role in women as well; especially around ovulation. It supports confidence, libido, and muscle growth.

The natural ebb and flow of these hormones over the course of your cycle creates four distinct phases, each with its own strengths, challenges, and needs. Let's explore them.

The 4 Phases of the Menstrual Cycle

Your cycle typically runs 24–35 days and has four phases, each with unique hormonal shifts that influence how you feel and function.

Phase 1: Menstrual (Days 1–5)

This is the phase when your period starts: Day 1 of your cycle. Technically the start of menstruation is the start of your follicular phase as well. Estrogen and progesterone are at their lowest levels, and your body is shedding the uterine lining it built up the previous month. You might feel low-energy, introverted, or even a little foggy. That's completely normal. This is your body's natural reset button.

Use this time to lean into rest, reflection, and gentle movement. Think walks, stretching, restorative yoga anything that feels nourishing instead of depleting. Warm, iron-rich foods like soups, lentils, and leafy greens can help replenish lost nutrients.

> **Journal prompt:** What does rest look like for me right now? What do I need to let go of?

Phase 2: Follicular (Days 1–13)

As your period ends, estrogen begins to rise and your body starts preparing for ovulation. The follicles in your ovaries mature, and your brain and body gradually shift out of rest-and-recovery mode. Most women notice a natural upswing in energy, mood, and mental clarity during this phase.

This is a great time to lean into more structured workouts, strength training, or learning new skills. Your body is primed for progress, and your mind is often more focused and adventurous. From a nutrition standpoint, lighter, protein-rich meals and fiber-rich foods can support your metabolism and gut health. You may also find yourself more socially engaged or creatively inspired during this window. Use this energy to brainstorm, plan, or action new ideas.

> 📝 **Journal prompt:** What challenge am I excited to take on this week? What new habit do I want to try?

Phase 3: Ovulatory (Around Day 14)

This is your peak window. Estrogen levels surge, and your body releases an egg in anticipation of fertilization. A small boost of testosterone kicks in and gives you a noticeable edge in energy, strength, and confidence. Many women feel their most vibrant and outgoing during this time.

Physically, this is a great phase for challenging workouts like high intensity interval training (HIIT), powerlifting, or any type of group class where you're feeding off high energy. Mentally and emotionally, it's an ideal time for collaboration, connection, and communicating your ideas. To support this high-energy window, focus on fresh produce, hydration, and high-quality protein to fuel your performance.

> **Journal prompt:** What makes me feel most powerful right now? How can I show up fully this week?

Phase 4: Luteal (Days 15–28)

After ovulation, progesterone rises and estrogen starts to decline. This shift prepares your body for a potential pregnancy, and if one doesn't occur, you'll begin the hormonal descent into your next menstrual phase. The luteal phase can feel like a slow wind-down: energy begins to dip, and your body asks for more rest and grounding.

You might notice increased sensitivity, cravings, or trouble sleeping, especially in the late luteal days right before your period. Instead of pushing through with intense workouts, this is the time to prioritize steady-state cardio, lower-impact strength sessions, or extra rest. Support your mood and recovery with magnesium-rich foods like pumpkin seeds, leafy greens, and yes, dark chocolate. It's a good time to review your boundaries and build in extra space for self-care.

> 📝 **Journal prompt:** What do I need more of, and less of, this week? Where can I build in softness?

How Women's Physiology Differs from Men's: Why It Matters

If you read the previous section about the four phases of the menstrual cycle, you already know that the female body runs on a very different rhythm than the male body. While men operate on a relatively stable 24-hour hormonal cycle (Think: consistent testosterone levels day to day) women move through a multi-phase, monthly cycle where key hormones rise and fall dramatically. For most of modern history, scientific research, medical guidelines, and fitness advice were based on one default subject: the average young, healthy male. It was simpler and easier to control variables; but it also ignored half the population.

Women's bodies aren't just smaller versions of men's. They operate on a different biological rhythm that is governed by hormones that fluctuate across the month and a woman's lifetime. These fluctuations affect how we train, what we crave, how we recover, how we sleep, and how we respond to stress. Ignoring this isn't just unfair, it's ineffective.

Compared to men, women generally burn more fat and fewer carbohydrates during low- to moderate-intensity exercise. This is influenced by estrogen, which promotes lipid oxidation (the conversion of fat into energy). Women experience more pronounced metabolic disruptions in response to caloric restriction or overtraining which can lead to menstrual dysfunction or energy deficiency.

Recent research shows that women gain strength and muscle mass at comparable rates to men when training consistently but women start with less absolute muscle mass. This makes resistance training especially important as a tool to preserve muscle and bone density, particularly during and after menopause when estrogen declines.

The female stress response is also distinct. Because women have a more reactive hypothalamic-pituitary-adrenal (HPA) axis, they may experience and internalize stress differently than men. Chronic stress, paired with fluctuating progesterone and estrogen levels, can further dysregulate mood, energy, and sleep cycles.

When it comes to sleep, women are more likely to experience sleep disturbances, particularly during the luteal phase of the cycle, in the postpartum period, and throughout perimenopause. Disrupted sleep contributes to poor recovery, increased appetite, and a decrease in overall resilience.

These physiological differences don't mean that we need special treatment. It means we need accurate information, and appropriate strategies. When we honor how the female body actually works, we stop blaming ourselves for "inconsistency" or "lack of willpower," and start creating strategies that align with our biology. That's where real, lasting change begins.

CHAPTER 2
HOW HABITS REALLY WORK

Once we understand how the female body changes throughout the month, we can begin to build habits that actually work with that rhythm instead of against it.

Most traditional habit advice is built around the idea that consistency means doing the same thing every day. Same time, same way, no matter what. But life in a female body doesn't work like that. Energy levels shift. Sleep changes. Cravings ebb and flow. Some days you're on fire; other days, making coffee feels like a full-body workout.

This isn't failure. This is being in rhythm and the more you understand your own rhythm, the better your habits can support you long term.

Rethinking "Consistency"

Let's say you've decided to work out four times a week. Week one goes great! You've got the energy, your schedule's manageable, and it feels good to move your body. Week two hits, and suddenly you're more tired, your cravings are up, and your calendar looks like a Tetris board of appointments and responsibilities. Maybe you're in the luteal phase of your cycle, or maybe life just got heavier that week. You miss two workouts, feel frustrated, and start questioning whether you're cut out for this.

This is where most habit-building falls apart, not because people don't care enough or lack motivation, but because we expect consistency to look the same all the time. It doesn't. And it shouldn't.

A better approach is to think of consistency like a rhythm, something you return to, but not always with the same intensity. One of my clients started using a color-coded system to track her workouts: green days were full sessions, yellow days meant shortened or low-impact movement, and red days were intentional rest. She noticed that during "off" weeks, she was still showing up. She wasn't pushing herself to do the exact same thing every day, but she kept the habit alive in a way that honored how she felt. That simple shift, recognizing that a walk counts, that stretching matters, helped her stay consistent for months, not just a week or two.

Consistency isn't about repeating the same action over and over. It's staying connected to the intention behind the action and being willing to adapt.

Most women never hear: your body isn't the same from week to week. So, if you're tracking progress; whether it's weight, strength, mood, or energy; the most accurate way to measure it is by comparing where you are in your cycle.

Personally, I never compare a client's weight week to week. We only compare it at the same point in their cycle. Your weight today should be compared to your weight on the same day of your last cycle, not last Tuesday. Why? Because during your luteal phase, you might be retaining more water. During menstruation, your energy might be lower. During ovulation, you might feel like a superhero. Progress isn't linear, it's cyclical. And when you start viewing it that way, the whole game changes. You stop obsessing over fluctuations, and you start understanding your patterns.

This is why rhythm matters more than routine. You don't need to hit the same numbers every day, you just need to stay in tune with your body and your life.

Why Small Wins Work Better than Big Overhauls

Most people think that if you really want to change your life, you have to go all in. Start a new diet, overhaul your training plan, wake up at 5 a.m., cut sugar, cut screens, cut fun. It's intense, and let's be real, it's usually short-lived!

What happens when you get sick? Or your kid's daycare closes? Or you hit your luteal phase and feel like curling up in a blanket burrito instead of meal prepping quinoa and broccoli?

That's when the big-overhaul approach starts to crack. Not because you aren't disciplined, but because it wasn't built for real life.

Small wins, on the other hand, keep the momentum going when things get unpredictable. I had a client who told me she didn't work out at all for one week and was beating herself up over it. But when we looked closer, we saw that she walked her dog every morning, chose a protein-rich snack instead of skipping lunch, and stretched for five minutes before bed. That's not failure, that's exactly what we'd been working toward: stacking sustainable actions that fit into the actual rhythm of her life.

These moments build self-trust. They show your brain, "Hey, I show up, even when things aren't perfect." And that's the magic. You're not striving for perfection, you're trying to build a pattern that supports you through *everything*, not just the easy weeks.

Over time, these small wins become your foundation. They aren't flashy, but they're sustainable. They create space for real change that sticks, not just change that looks good for a week on Instagram.

Compassion Over Criticism

Women are good at being hard on themselves. We've been raised to believe that if we do not push harder, strive more, or improve constantly, we fall behind. Here's what took me decades to learn: the real fuel for progress isn't pressure, it's compassion.

Self-compassion does not let yourself off the hook. Remove the hook entirely. Recognize that being human: messy, hormonal, sleep-deprived, overstretched, isn't something to fix. It's something to support.

When you treat yourself like someone worth caring for, everything changes. You come back to your habits faster. You recover from setbacks more easily. And you stop seeing every detour as a disaster.

Habits That Match Your Life

Your habits don't need to look like anyone else's. They don't need to be perfect. They don't need to be polished or posted. They just need to feel good for you.

Habits that work over the long haul are built from a foundation of flexibility, rhythm, and self-respect. They honor your biology. They account for your real-life schedule. They leave room for rest, softness, and joy, not just hustle.

If you've ever felt like you "just can't stick with things," you just haven't found the habits that work for you yet.

Stop forcing rigid routines onto ever-changing bodies. Start building systems that breathe with us. Let's create habits that make space for the full spectrum of who we are: strong, tired, motivated, emotional, soft, focused, scattered, powerful.

All of it belongs. And all of it counts.

CHAPTER 3
THE PILLARS OF WELLNESS

In today's world, being healthy can feel way more complicated than it needs to be. A constant stream of wellness trends, cold plunges, detox teas, biohacking gadgets,and endless supplements, promise to be the thing that will change your life. One day it's intermittent fasting, the next it's six meals a day. These so-called "health hacks" might have some benefits, but they've also made the basics feel unclear and overwhelming.

And as much as I love cold plunging, the truth is, you don't need to hack your health. You need to support it. At its core, wellness isn't built on extremes or trends; it's grounded in four foundational pillars that hold everything together: movement, nourishment, rest, and recovery. These aren't flashy, but they're powerful. When they're in balance, they make everything else simpler.

I want to stress the importance that these pillars aren't just things to "check off" your to-do list; they're foundational practices that influence how your body functions, how your mind feels, and how you show up in your daily life. When one pillar is off, the others are affected., When you start to care for all of them simultaneously, even in small ways, you create a stable foundation that real change can be built on.

Keep in mind that these pillars won't always look the same week to week or from one phase of life to another. It's important to learn how to tune in and adjust to your current needs.

How do these pillars actually work in real life? That's where things start to feel a lot more manageable, and a lot less intimidating.

Note: *What you're about to read is a big-picture look at the four foundational pillars of wellness. We'll explore how each of these pillars can be adapted and optimized for different life stages, like puberty, reproductive years, perimenopause, and post-menopause, later in the book. You don't need to figure it all out now. For now, start to notice how these areas show up in your daily life.*

Movement

Movement should be a love letter to your body, not a punishment for what you ate or a chore to earn your rest. Whether it's lifting heavy, dancing around your kitchen, hiking, swimming, walking your dog, or doing ten squats between meetings, it all counts. The key is consistency and variety, not perfection.

Strength training is especially important for women because we naturally carry less muscle mass than men, and we start to lose it earlier than most people realize. In fact, age-related muscle loss, called sarcopenia, can begin as early as your 30s. It's valuable to build up as much muscle mass and strength as possible *before* menopause, when the rate of muscle and bone loss accelerates. Lifting weights isn't just about aesthetics, it's about setting yourself up for long-term function, resilience, and independence. It preserves bone density, improves insulin sensitivity, supports metabolic health, and builds confidence: not just in how you look, but in how capable you feel.

Your body responds differently to movement depending on where you are in your cycle. You might feel energized and ready to push during your follicular and ovulatory phases, while your luteal and menstrual phases may call for lower-impact movement or more rest. Listening to those shifts isn't lazy: it's *smart programming*. We will go in depth into this in chapter 7.

If you're in a life phase where high-intensity anything feels like too much (early postpartum, perimenopause, a season of burnout), scale back without guilt. Go for walks. Do mobility work. Stretch. Movement doesn't have to mean sweat, it just means *motion*.

Motion is lotion.

Nutrition

Food should fuel, nourish, and support; not confuse, shame, or restrict. So many women have been taught to approach nutrition through the lens of fear: don't eat carbs, don't eat after 6 p.m., don't eat "too much." But the truth is, eating *enough* of the right nutrients, at the right times, is one of the most powerful forms of self-care you can practice.

Women's nutritional needs fluctuate throughout the month, and your body constantly communicates what it needs. Crave more carbs during your luteal phase? Your body is asking for accessible energy to support increased metabolic demand. Craving salt or chocolate during menstruation? Your body is nudging you to replenish magnesium and iron.

The more you learn to listen, and respond without judgment, the more balanced and supported you'll feel. Build your meals around protein, fiber, and healthy fats and adjust portions and timing based on your energy, activity level, and cycle phase.

Let's drop the "perfect diet" myth. It's not about being flawless. We want a flexible, sustainable approach to eating that makes you feel good and gives your body what it needs to thrive.

Rest (Sleep)

Without quality sleep, everything else suffers. Your hormones get thrown off. Your hunger cues go haywire. Your ability to think clearly, handle stress, and make healthy choices all take a hit.

The challenge? Many women, especially in the luteal phase, postpartum, or perimenopause, struggle to get solid, uninterrupted sleep. Hormonal shifts can make it harder to fall asleep, stay asleep, or feel rested in the morning. Add in stress, parenting, or racing thoughts at 3 a.m., and it's no wonder so many women feel depleted.

Instead of trying to "hack" sleep with supplements or apps, start with the basics:

- Prioritize a consistent bedtime

- Limit screen time before bed

- Create a calming wind-down routine

- Eat enough throughout the day to avoid blood sugar crashes overnight

Don't treat sleep like a luxury. It's a biological necessity, not an optional add-on. If you're struggling with energy, mood, or motivation, look at your sleep. It's often the missing piece.

Recovery (Regulate)

Recovery is the pillar that I find most women intentionally skip. Not because they don't want it, but because they don't think they're "allowed." We live in a culture that celebrates hustle and productivity, but your body doesn't build strength, resilience, or hormonal balance during *the work*. It builds it during *the recovery*. The work is the stimulus for the adaptation to occur. Without allowing your body a chance to recover, you're denying her the chance to adapt.

Recovery includes everything from active rest days to stress management, nervous system regulation, and emotional processing. It's taking a few deep breaths after a long meeting. It's giving yourself permission to not "power through" when you're fried. It's understanding the difference between being tired from training and tired from life.

Recovery shifts with your hormones. During your luteal phase, your nervous system becomes more sensitive to stress. During perimenopause, you might find your tolerance for overstimulation drops.

Building in more deliberate recovery practices, like breathwork, nature therapy, quiet time, or gentle movement, helps your body reset.

One of my favorite reminders: *motion is lotion, but stillness is medicine*. You need both.

Tailoring Your Pillars to You

These four pillars, movement, nutrition, rest, and recovery, are the foundations of sustainable wellness. How you should approach each one will shift based on your season of life, your current energy, your goals, and your phase of the cycle.

There will be weeks when you hit the gym four times and feel amazing. There will be weeks when the biggest win is going for a walk and eating a warm, nourishing meal. Both are valid and are part of the rhythm. What matters most isn't what you do perfectly, it's that you stay connected to your body, your values, and your ability to keep coming back.

Wellness doesn't mean you need to maximize every minute of your day. It's about learning how to support your body where it's at, and giving it what it needs to thrive.

Build Your Pillar Plan

Use this worksheet to reflect on how each of the four wellness pillars - Movement, Nutrition, Sleep, and Recovery - currently fit into your life. This plan is not perfect. The goal is to tune into what you need right now and identify small, supportive shifts that align with your energy, goals, and life phase.

Movement

- What types of movement feel best in my body right now?

_____

_____

_____

- How many days a week would feel supportive, not stressful?

_____

_____

_____

- What is one way I can move more without adding pressure?

_____

_____

_____

Nutrition

- How do I feel before and after I eat most meals?

_____

_____

_____

- What is one meal I could make easier or more nourishing?

_____

_____

_____

- Where can I be more flexible or forgiving with my eating habits?

_____

_____

_____

Sleep

- How is my sleep quality lately?

_____

_____

_____

- What helps me wind down before bed?

_____
_____
_____

- What is one thing I can shift this week to protect my rest?

_____
_____
_____

Recovery

- What drains me the most right now - physically or emotionally?

_____
_____
_____

- What activities help me feel calm and grounded?

_____
_____
_____

- What boundary or habit could help me recover better this week?

_____

_____

_____

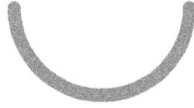

PART II
ADOLESCENCE & PUBERTY: THE EARLY YEARS

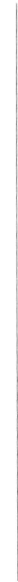

CHAPTER 4
WHERE IT ALL BEGAN

If you're anything like me, nobody handed you a guidebook for puberty. We learned the basics: periods, pregnancy, maybe a few awkward facts in health class, but not how our hormones would shape our energy, moods, and sense of self. Maybe someone gave you a book to read, or maybe it was just whispered advice from a friend. But real, honest conversations about what was happening inside our bodies? Those were rare.

What we didn't realize back then is that puberty wasn't just chaos, it was construction. Those early years were the start of a lifelong relationship with your body. Every change, every surge of emotion, every new boundary was laying the groundwork for how you'd learn to take care of yourself. The habits you formed, the way you talked to yourself, even how you handled stress or rest, all of it started there.

You weren't just surviving puberty. You were building the foundation for everything that would come next.

You Were Going Through a Full-Body Renovation

Looking back, it's no wonder it felt overwhelming. Your hormones, estrogen, progesterone, testosterone, were rapidly changing, sending ripples through every system in your body.

Remember some of these milestones?

- Growing taller almost overnight

- Developing breasts and hips

- Getting your first period (whether you were ready for it or not)

- Skin changes that made mirrors uncomfortable

- Emotional rollercoasters that showed up out of nowhere

- Feeling wired at night and exhausted by morning

And then came the social layer: suddenly, you became aware of how others saw you. You started noticing your reflection more, comparing yourself to friends, to media, to impossible beauty standards. That shift wasn't "just in your head" it was also a neurological one. Studies show that girls' self-esteem often peaks *before* puberty and begins to decline during it. If that sounds familiar, you're not imagining it. The world got louder, and it became harder to feel at home in your own skin.

You Deserved to Be Taught How to Listen

Most of us were taught that our bodies were unpredictable and inconvenient, something to "deal with," not something to trust. What if, instead, someone had told you:

- Your hunger cues, mood shifts, and energy crashes: they're messages, not failures.

- Your period isn't an inconvenience: it's a vital sign of health.

- You're not "too emotional": you're responding to real, powerful hormonal changes.

That's body literacy. And if you didn't get that education back then, you're going to get it now!

Your body has always been talking to you. Learning to listen, and trust what you hear, is one of the most revolutionary habits you can build.

Movement Was Supposed to Be a Celebration

Think back: Did you love moving your body as a kid? Running around? Dancing without worrying how you looked? Swimming for hours?

Puberty hit and maybe things changed. You got self-conscious. You worried about how you looked in shorts or swimsuits. Maybe you dropped out of sports you used to love, not because you didn't want to move, but because suddenly, it felt different.

Here's what I wish every girl heard during puberty (and what I hope you hear now):

Movement:

- Is not a punishment
- Is not about earning food or fixing flaws.
- Is a love letter to your strength, resilience, and aliveness.
- It doesn't have to be a "sport" to count.
- Dancing around your room? Counts.
- Walking your dog? Counts.
- Trying a new sport and being hilariously bad at it? Definitely counts.

Movement builds *trust* in your body. It reminds you that you're powerful, especially in the moments when you forget.

Food Was Never Meant to Be the Enemy

Somewhere along the way, a lot of us got the message that food was something to fear: Don't eat too much, don't eat the wrong thing, don't *crave* anything.

But your body isn't wrong for wanting nourishment. She's wise.

Maybe you remember craving salty foods around your period, or feeling like you could eat everything in sight during certain times of the month. That wasn't you being "undisciplined", that was your metabolism shifting, your body asking for what it needed.

Sleep, Screens, and Stress: The New Normal

If puberty wasn't complicated enough, many of us also came of age during the rise of constant screens. Phones. Social media. Netflix. Gaming. And suddenly, getting enough sleep wasn't just about being tired, it was a daily battle against late-night scrolling, comparison traps, and the feeling of always being "on."

Remember:

- Staying up way later than you meant to.

- Waking up exhausted but still grabbing your phone first thing.

- Feeling wired, tired, and overwhelmed without knowing why.

If that pattern stuck with you, it wasn't because you were "bad at self-control." You adapted to a world that didn't respect your biology.

Sleep is the ultimate recovery tool, and even small shifts (like screen-free time before bed, or having a consistent bedtime) can change everything. We might not have the ability to go completely screen free before bed, but simple things like wearing blue light blocking glasses can help you to avoid some of the stimulating effects.

You Deserved Compassion Then. You Still Do Now.

Maybe the people around you didn't understand what you needed during puberty. Maybe you didn't understand either.

But you deserved compassion then and you deserve it now.

You deserved to know:

- That it was okay to be tired, hungry, moody, changing.
- That your body was doing exactly what it was supposed to do.
- That you didn't have to fight yourself to be worthy.

Puberty wasn't the beginning of problems. It was the beginning of your resilience, your adaptability, and your ability to thrive through change. And now, as we move forward, you get to keep building on that foundation, with more trust, more wisdom, and way more compassion for everything you've already survived.

The habits you formed back then, whether by design or by survival, still echo in how you move, eat, rest, and recover today. Now it's time to take a closer look at those core areas of wellness. Not to pick apart what you're doing wrong, but to reconnect with what your body has always been asking for and to start building habits that truly support the woman you're becoming.

CHAPTER 5
FOUNDATIONS FOR LIFE

When you think back to your teen years, you might realize how many of your current habits first took root without you even noticing. Some habits you probably carried forward intentionally, others just happened. They were shaped by what you knew at the time, what you had access to, and what the people around you modeled.

Our teenage years shouldn't be just about surviving high school and hormones. This is the phase where we are building our foundational habits and building a strong base that we can build our mansions on.

Creating Healthy Habits That Stick into Adulthood

Healthy habits don't magically appear when you turn thirty, forty, or fifty. They start earlier, often in ways you didn't even realize were happening. If you were praised for skipping meals or eating very little, you might have learned to ignore your hunger cues. If you were pushed to overtrain in sports without rest, you might have internalized the idea that movement is supposed to be a punishment instead of a celebration. If you were only celebrated for achievements, high grades, athletic wins, looking a certain way, you might have learned to value productivity over health, or appearance over how you actually felt.

Even if the habits you built back then weren't ideal for your long-term health, you are never stuck with them. Habits aren't fixed traits; they're patterns you can understand, adjust, and rewire. And the more compassion you bring to that process, the easier it becomes. You're not starting from scratch: you're building on all the lessons your body has been trying to teach you from the very beginning.

Sleep, Screen Time, and Stress Management in the Teen Years

Looking back, you might remember how different your energy felt during those early years. You probably needed a lot more sleep than you were getting and not just because of school schedules or late-night texting marathons. Biologically, teenagers are wired to have a later sleep-wake cycle. Your natural rhythm likely shifted forward by a couple of hours, meaning you felt most awake later at night and struggled with early mornings.

Sleep

If no one explained that to you, you might have blamed yourself for feeling lazy, unmotivated, or exhausted. But your body wasn't failing you, it was doing exactly what it was programmed to do. And the consequences of chronic sleep deprivation at that age often ripple forward: difficulty to manage stress, struggle with focus and memory, and changes to appetite and metabolism. Learn to prioritize sleep, even in small ways, it isn't just important for teenagers, it's a skill we carry into adulthood, and one that many women end up circling back to later when burnout forces them to reconsider their priorities.

Screen Time

Most of us didn't grow up with an instruction manual for how to coexist with technology. Phones, social media, and streaming services crept into our lives, and before we realized it, they became part of our default rhythms: scrolling late at night, comparing ourselves to impossible images, feeling overstimulated without understanding why. Screens aren't evil. They're powerful tools, but they require boundaries. And like any other habit, setting healthy limits around screen time isn't about restriction; it's about protecting your energy, your nervous system, and your ability to be fully present in your own life.

Stress

Whether it showed up as school pressure, sports expectations, family dynamics, or social drama, stress in the teen years taught you something about how you cope under pressure. Did you learn to power through or shut down? Did you turn to food, numbing behaviors, or perfectionism to feel in control? None of those coping strategies were wrong, they were survival skills. But if they've followed you into adulthood in ways that don't feel helpful anymore, now is the time to update them. Breathwork, movement, journaling, quiet time in nature, therapy, hese aren't luxuries. They're necessary tools for managing the realities of a full, demanding life.

Supporting Girls with Compassion (And Reparenting Ourselves!)

If you were lucky enough to have parents, coaches, or mentors who supported you with compassion during your teen years, you know how powerful that steady presence can be. But not everyone had that. Maybe you were pushed instead of supported. Critiqued instead of celebrated. Ignored when you needed someone to simply listen.

If that resonates with you, here's something important: you can give yourself now what you didn't always get then. You can reparent the parts of you that needed gentleness, patience, and understanding. It starts with recognizing that health habits aren't a punishment for who you used to be, they're a gift for the woman you're becoming.

If you're in a role now where you support teenage girls, whether as a parent, coach, teacher, or mentor, you have an opportunity to help build a different foundation. One based on trust, not fear. One where rest is respected, nourishment is celebrated, and self-worth isn't tied to performance or appearance.

The goal isn't to raise perfect girls. It's to raise girls who trust their bodies, understand their rhythms, and know how to take care of themselves from a place of respect, not resentment.

And honestly? That's the same goal for us, too.

The habits you started to build in your early years, whether intentionally or by default, became the foundation you carried into adulthood. But as you moved out of adolescence and into your reproductive years, your body didn't just settle down and stay the same. It evolved, cycling through changes every single month, whether you realized it or not.

Understanding those rhythms, and learning to work with them instead of against them, is one of the most powerful ways to deepen your connection to your body. In Part 3, we'll explore how your hormones shape everything from your energy to your mood to your motivation and how syncing your habits with your natural cycle can change the game for your health, your confidence, and your life.

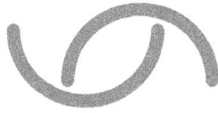

PART III
THE REPRODUCTIVE YEARS : CYCLE SYNCING AND THRIVING

CHAPTER 6
CYCLE SYNCING AND THRIVING

A rhythm pulses through your body every single month: a rhythm that influences your energy, your motivation, your cravings, your sleep, your performance, and your emotions. For years, I didn't know this. I treated my body like it should perform the same way every day. I blamed myself if I felt tired or heavy. I assumed low-energy days were a character flaw, not a biological reality.

It wasn't until about five years ago, when I committed to learning about my cycle and actually living *with* it instead of against it, that everything started to make sense. Now, I build my routines, including the writing of this book, around the natural ebbs and flows of my cycle. I write during my follicular phase, when creativity flows easily. I train hardest when my energy is highest, and I lean into mobility, active recovery, and reflection when my body signals that it's time to slow down.

Learning to live in sync with your cycle doesn't mean

you do less. It means you *strategize better*. It means you learn to trust your body's wisdom, and you stop seeing natural fluctuations as failures. When you listen, your body will tell you exactly what she needs.

The Four Phases of Your Cycle

Every month, whether you're fully aware of it or not, your body cycles through four distinct phases: menstrual, follicular, ovulatory and luteal.

Each phase comes with its own hormonal landscape, and each landscape shapes how you train, eat, sleep, recover, and feel.

The **follicular phase** begins on the first day of your period and stretches until ovulation. Even though you're bleeding at the start of this phase, your body is actually revving up for renewal. Estrogen levels start low but climb steadily, bringing with them a sense of lightness, energy, and focus. You might notice you feel more social, more willing to try new things, and more excited to tackle challenges. Training often feels easier here, your body responds well to progressive overload, new skills, and a bit of a push. Nutrition-wise, your appetite may feel a little lower and digestion more efficient. Sleep tends to be deep and refreshing, and motivation feels natural rather than forced. This is the perfect time to dream bigger, plan your projects, try new movements, and ride the wave of possibility. As I write these words, I'm deep in my follicular phase, and I can feel that familiar buzz. the creative energy, the quickness of thought, the willingness to push. Harnessing this phase is like planting seeds in fresh, fertile ground.

As you transition into the **ovulatory phase**, typically around the middle of your cycle, estrogen peaks and your body prepares to release an egg. Testosterone gets a little bump too, and suddenly, you feel powerful, magnetic, and capable. This is often the phase where strength, speed, and endurance hit their highest points. You recover faster, lift heavier, and move with more ease. Outside of training, your communication skills sharpen, your confidence rises, and you naturally gravitate toward collaboration and connection. Food cravings might increase slightly as your metabolism picks up, but overall, you feel steady and strong. Sleep tends to stay solid as long as you manage stress well. This is your body's "summertime" and everything is vibrant, alive, ready to perform. It's a beautiful time to hit personal records, have important conversations, or step into leadership roles.

And then, the **luteal phase** begins, the most complex phase of the cycle. After ovulation, your body starts preparing for the possibility of pregnancy, even if you're not trying to conceive. Progesterone rises, estrogen drops off, and with those shifts, you may notice subtle (or not-so-subtle) changes. Your energy begins to slow. Workouts feel heavier. You might crave more carbohydrates, salt, and chocolate. Sleep becomes more fragile; you might fall asleep later or wake up feeling less refreshed. Emotionally, sensitivity often rises. It's not all bad: this phase can bring incredible attention to detail, deeper reflection, and powerful intuition. But physically, it's common to feel less bulletproof.

I didn't understand any of this when I was a teenager, which made certain experiences even harder than they needed to be. I remember one swim practice vividly. I was about fourteen or fifteen. Our coach had set up a timed 400-meter swim. The instructions were clear: if he thought you didn't try hard enough, you had to redo it. I remember diving in, arms and legs heavy, my whole body sluggish. No matter how badly I *wanted* to swim fast, I couldn't access the extra gear. When the times were called out, I was one of the swimmers who had to get back on the block. As I bent down into position for the second attempt, tears welled up in my eyes. I dove in, crying before my face even hit the water, and sobbed silently through the entire 400 meters. My second time was even slower than my first. Afterward, my coach pulled me aside and apologized, he could see it wasn't laziness. My body had simply hit a wall. I didn't know it then, but looking back now, I would bet almost anything that I was deep into my luteal phase.

That story reminds me why understanding our cycle matters, not so we can opt out of challenges, but so we can meet ourselves with compassion. If you're a competitive athlete, you don't always get the luxury of adjusting. Sometimes you have to perform no matter what phase you're in. But knowing where you are gives you the power to support yourself better, by fueling differently, warming up longer, managing expectations, or doubling down on recovery afterward. Cycle syncing isn't about being fragile. It's about being informed. It's about using every tool available to work smarter, not harder.

Finally, the **menstrual phase** arrives. When your period starts, both estrogen and progesterone crash to their lowest levels. Your body is clearing out and resetting. It's normal during this time to feel lower in energy, heavier in your body, and more drawn to rest. Inflammation markers increase slightly, which can make soreness or fatigue more noticeable. Sleep needs can rise, and your appetite might swing depending on how your body handles hormonal shifts. It's a natural time for slowing down, not necessarily stopping everything, but choosing more restorative movement: walks, stretching, mobility, or lighter strength work if you feel up to it.

Contrary to popular belief, your period is not a sign of weakness. It's a built-in recovery system, a natural reset that helps your body prepare for another month of possibility.

What the Research Says (and What It Misses)

Now, you might have heard some skepticism about cycle syncing. And it's true: research doesn't consistently show significant differences in maximal strength output across different phases of the cycle. Some studies report no meaningful change in how much weight you can lift or how hard you can push.

But what that research often misses is the *lived experience* of women. It doesn't always capture the increased perception of effort during the luteal phase. It doesn't track the cumulative effects of poorer sleep, higher inflammation, and emotional load. It doesn't quantify the quiet fatigue that builds when you're pushing through hormonal headwinds.

If I complete twelve quality training sessions over a month by doing four workouts per week for three weeks, and then taking a week to focus on active recovery, that's still twelve sessions. The volume stays the same. The effort stays high. I'm just organizing my effort more efficiently, in a way that honors my biology. It's no different than someone training three times a week steadily for four weeks. but it feels dramatically better, and my body adapts more easily.

Cycle syncing isn't about *doing less*. It's about *doing smarter*.

Learning to Flow with It

By now you should start to see that your cycle isn't something to be conquered or overcome. It's a map that needs to be read. And when you learn to read it, you unlock more freedom, not less.

Instead of beating yourself up for feeling slower during your luteal phase, you can adjust your training, nutrition, and recovery and still stay consistent. Instead of forcing yourself to perform at peak intensity every single day, you can lean into your natural highs and respect your natural lows.

You don't have to be perfect. You just have to be willing to listen, to work *with* your body instead of constantly fighting her. This is the beginning of real strength. The kind that doesn't just come from lifting heavier weights or hitting faster splits, but from learning how to support yourself, inside and out.

Track to Thrive

If you've made it this far, I hope you are starting to shift the way you think about your cycle, and maybe, about yourself. You're no longer seeing your hormonal changes as obstacles. You're beginning to see them as *information*. Signals. Feedback. A roadmap for how to take better care of yourself.

But knowing your phases is just the beginning. Real magic happens when you notice how *you* feel through each part of your cycle. Not the textbook version. Not someone else's story. Yours.

That's where tracking comes in.

This doesn't need to be complicated. You don't need fancy apps or a dozen data points. Just a few quick notes each day:

- How you slept.

- What your energy felt like.

- Any mood shifts or physical sensations.

- How your workouts went (or didn't).

- What you craved, what helped, what didn't.

The goal isn't to control every variable. It's to notice patterns. Over time, you'll begin to recognize your own rhythm: when you feel strongest, when you need rest, when to push, and when to pull back.

You'll also start to see your symptoms in a new light: bloating, brain fog, cravings, fatigue. These aren't random. They're clues. And the more awareness you bring, the more you can support your body with food, movement, rest, and grace.

The next page includes a simple monthly tracker. Use it however you like: daily, weekly, or just during key moments. There's no wrong way to do it, only your way.

This is the beginning of a deeper relationship with your body. One built on trust, not punishment. One rooted in curiosity, not shame. One that evolves, just like you do.

You're not meant to be the same every day.

But you *are* meant to feel at home in your body.

Let's start there.

Monthly Cycle Tracker

Track physical, emotional, and energetic shifts across your cycle

Day	Physical Notes	Mood/Energy	Cycle Phase
1			
2			
3			
4			
5			
6			
7			
8			
9			
10			
11			
12			
13			
14			
15			
16			
17			
18			
19			
20			
21			
22			
23			
24			
25			
26			
27			
28			
29			
30			
31			

CHAPTER 7
LIVING IN SYNC

Understanding your individual cycle is a powerful tool. But applying that understanding to real life? That's where everything changes.

It's one thing to know that your energy will shift through the month. It's another thing to *work with it*, adjust your workouts, your nutrition, your expectations, and your self-talk so that you stay consistent, but flexible. This chapter is about taking what you learned and putting it into practice in a way that feels sustainable, empowering, and totally doable in real life, not just in theory. The goal isn't to obsess over every hormonal fluctuation or treat yourself like a science experiment. The goal is to become so deeply connected to your own rhythms that you naturally know when to push, when to ease off, when to fuel differently, and when to rest without guilt.

One of my clients, Talia, really lives this. In her late 20s, she came to me wanting to feel more energized and consistent in her workouts. Like so many women, she spent years thinking her fluctuating energy was a personal flaw, something she needed to push through or fix with more discipline. But once we started tracking her cycle and connecting it to her training, she began noticing clear patterns.

Her energy surged during her follicular and ovulatory phases, so we loaded her heavier strength work, HIIT, and high-performance sessions into those weeks. She also started noticing the impact beyond the gym. When she could choose, she booked important meetings, speaking engagements, and creative brainstorming sessions during those phases, when she felt confident, outgoing, and sharp. During her luteal phase, she blocked off time to tie up loose ends, finalize reports, and focus on detail-heavy work. She leaned into what her body naturally wanted to do... and it worked!

When her cycle moved into the menstrual phase, we shifted her workouts accordingly. She focused on recovery, lighter lifting, walking, and mobility. This wasn't because she needed to back off, but because she learned how to train smart and respect what her body needed.

After a few months, Talia stopped blaming herself for the off days. She no longer forced herself to push through just to check a box. She recognized her body's signals and used them to her advantage. Her progress picked up. Her mindset softened. Her self-trust deepened.

She no longer needed an app or tracker to tell her what to do. She could feel when to push and when to pause. That's the power of syncing with your body, not obsessing over the details. It is a beautiful thing knowing yourself so well, that flowing with your rhythm becomes second nature.

Adjusting Your Workouts Across the Month

You don't need four completely different training programs for each week of your cycle. Living in sync is about tweaking, not overhauling.

During your follicular and ovulatory phases, when estrogen is rising and peaking, your body is primed for building strength, speed, and endurance. This is the best window to go after heavier lifts, higher intensity workouts, and skill progression. Your recovery will likely be faster, your energy will feel higher, and you'll be more resilient to physical stress.

As you shift into the luteal phase, your nervous system becomes a little more sensitive. You might notice that high-intensity intervals feel harder, that your joints feel stiffer, or that your mental sharpness drops. This doesn't mean you should stop training; but it suggests that adjusting your approach could be a good idea. Think moderate weights, more steady-state cardio, longer warm-ups, and a greater emphasis on mobility, breathwork, or technique refinement. Support your body through a changing internal landscape instead of completely abandoning your goals.

When your period starts, give yourself permission to lead with how you feel. Some women feel better to move gently, walk, stretch, doing mobility flows, while others regain energy by day two or three and want to jump back into more structured training. Neither is wrong. Tune in and respect what your body is asking for, rather than forcing yourself to do what someone else is telling you to do.

The key principle to remember: consistency over intensity. Adjusting your intensity across the month keeps you consistent long-term. Consistency builds results faster than the occasional heroic effort does

Adjust Your Nutrition Across the Month

Just like your training needs shift, so do your nutrition needs. Learning to adjust the way you fuel yourself makes a massive difference in how you feel, recover, and perform across the month.

During your follicular phase (Days 1-14), when insulin sensitivity is higher and metabolism is steady, you might find that lighter meals with plenty of protein, healthy fats, fiber, and colorful carbs feel energizing and sustaining. Digestion is often smoother during this time, and you may naturally feel less hungry.

As ovulation approaches, your metabolism subtly ramps up. You might feel a little hungrier, and that's normal. Lean into increasing your caloric intake, especially around workouts and focus on balanced meals that keep blood sugar stable.

The luteal phase often brings the biggest changes. Progesterone increases your metabolic rate and can drive up hunger, cravings, and emotional eating tendencies. Instead of fighting it or labeling it as "bad," honor it by adjusting your meals: slightly larger portions, more satisfying carbohydrates (especially slow-digesting carbs like oats, sweet potatoes, rice), plenty of magnesium-rich foods (like leafy greens and dark chocolate), and making sure you're not skimping on calories overall. Under fueling during this phase almost always backfires with worse cravings, mood swings, and energy crashes.

During your period, cravings often shift again. You might crave warm, comforting foods like stews, soups, warm grains, and hearty meals which are perfectly aligned with your body's need for restoration. Focus on easy-to-digest, nourishing meals and adequate hydration to support recovery.

Let's walk through a real-world example to show how your calorie needs shift across the month:

Say your resting energy expenditure (REE), the number of calories your body burns at rest, is around 2,000 calories per day during the follicular phase. As you approach ovulation, your metabolism ramps up slightly. Research suggests that REE can increase by about 5% during this time, nudging your daily needs closer to 2,100 calories.

Then comes the luteal phase where things start to heat up, metabolically speaking. Thanks to rising progesterone levels, your body works a little harder behind the scenes. In the mid-to-late luteal phase, especially the week before your period, REE can rise by another 5%. That bumps your daily calorie needs up again, now you're closer to 2,200 calories per day.

That's an extra 200 calories per day compared to the start of your cycle, just from your body doing its usual hormone dance.

Cycle syncing your nutrition doesn't mean you need a different meal plan for each week of the month. During my period I always crave red meat, and I eat a lot of it during this week. The remainder of my follicular phase generally consists of salads and proteins. During my luteal phase I find myself wanting warm comforting foods so typically have more hearty, warm meals during this time. Listening to the natural shifts in my appetite and metabolism through the month keeps my diet varied, and decision fatigue (of what to eat) low!

Adjusting Your Expectations Across the Month

This might be the most important adjustment of all.

Stop measuring your worth by how perfectly you nail every workout or eat every meal. You're not a machine. You are a cyclical, dynamic human being. Some weeks, you are going to crush your to-do list and hit new PRs in the gym. Other weeks, you might count it as a win if you get out for a walk and eat something nourishing.

For me, living in sync doesn't mean lowering my standards, it means redefining what success looks like based on what my body actually needs, not some fantasy of constant, linear progress. I know my luteal phase tends to bring more fatigue and emotional sensitivity, so I shift my goals during that time. Maybe I schedule a reload (recovery) week in training. Maybe I tackle my most important work earlier in my cycle and leave the admin tasks for later.

When I stop expecting myself to be the same every day, I open the door to deeper consistency, better results, more peace.

Birth Control and Irregular Cycles?

If you're on hormonal birth control like the pill, hormonal IUD, implant, or patch; your natural cycle is largely overridden by synthetic hormones. You might not experience the same distinct rises and falls in estrogen and progesterone, which means your energy and mood might feel more stable, or sometimes flat. This doesn't mean you can't live in sync. You can still track your energy, mood, sleep, cravings, and recovery across the month and notice your personal patterns. Some women find they still experience a rhythm (even if it's less hormonally driven) tied to their placebo week or monthly cycles of life stress, training load, and recovery needs.

If you have irregular cycles, whether from Polycystic Ovary Syndrome (PCOS), perimenopause, recovery from birth control, stress, or another health condition, tracking becomes even more important, not less. Instead of tracking based only on bleeding days, focus on tracking daily symptoms: energy levels, sleep quality, mood, cravings, motivation, and how your body feels moving. Over time, you'll likely start to notice 'mini-patterns', even if your cycle isn't clockwork. And those patterns can help you guide your training, nutrition, and recovery strategies.

Living in sync with an irregular or medically managed cycle is all about paying attention to what's real for you.

Tracking Tips for Real Life

If you're just starting to track, keep it simple. Pick one or two things to notice each day. Maybe energy level and mood to start. Jot them down in a journal, your phone notes app, or use the Cycle Tracker provided in the previous chapter.

After a few months, patterns will start to emerge. You'll begin to see when you naturally feel your strongest, when cravings spike, when sleep gets rough, and when you need to pivot training or adjust nutrition. It is not about tracking every symptom perfectly, it's about developing a relationship with your body that's observant, compassionate, and responsive. You already have rhythms. Tracking just helps you see them more clearly, and live in partnership with them.

CHAPTER 8
POWER HABITS FOR THE
REPRODUCTIVE YEARS

Let's talk about stress. Because if there's one thing the reproductive years don't lack, it's pressure. There's the pressure to succeed at work. To be present in your relationship. To keep up with friends, maybe raise kids, definitely care for aging parents. The to-do list never ends, and for many women, that constant low-grade stress becomes the background music of their life.

But chronic stress doesn't just mess with your mood, it messes with everything. Your hormones, your sleep, your digestion, your ability to recover from workouts or even *enjoy* your downtime. The solution isn't a three-hour morning routine that involves green juice, cold plunges, journaling, sun-gazing, and meditating on a Himalayan rock- if that works for you GREAT! But most people don't have time for that. What you need are simple, doable strategies. Breathing deeply at a red light. Stretching while your coffee brews. Saying "no" more often without explaining yourself. Lying on the floor for five minutes in complete silence. These things matter. They don't look like much, but they shift the needle.

One of the most powerful things you can do in this chapter of life is learn to protect your energy, not just physically, but relationally. Some people in your life will give you energy and others will take it. You know the difference by how you feel after spending time with them. Drained? Dread-filled? Second-guessing yourself? Those are signs. You don't owe constant access to anyone. Boundaries are a form of self-care too.

And while we're here, let's talk about the relationship that matters most: *the one with yourself.*

There's a moment I have with almost every client, usually after a few weeks of working together. It's a quiet moment, often after a workout or during a check-in. They say something like, "I just don't recognize my body anymore." Or "I used to feel strong and now I just feel...tired." Or "I look in the mirror and I don't know who I am. If that's you, I want you to know: you're not alone. Your body changes during these years. It may not bounce back the way it used to. It might carry softness in new places. Your boobs might be a little less perky, your jeans might fit differently, your skin might show signs of stress or time or just life. Your body is not broken. It adapts. It Responds. It carries you.

What if instead of trying to force it back into some outdated mold, you got curious? What if you started paying attention, really paying attention, to what your body is trying to tell you? When are you most energized? When do you feel sluggish or bloated or wired? How do certain foods affect your mood or focus? What kind of movement leaves you feeling alive, not depleted? These are the breadcrumbs. Your body is always giving you feedback and you have to listen.

Making peace with your body isn't a one-time event. It's a practice. A muscle you build over time. The more you listen, the more you trust. The more you trust, the less you fight. And the less you fight, the more you get to live.

The reproductive years are busy, yes, but they're also a chance to build habits that will carry you into the next chapter. You don't have to do it all. You just have to do what matters most. And that starts with making space for you.

These years are often described as your "prime," but no one really talks about how exhausting that can feel. You're likely building a career, managing a home, maintaining relationships, maybe raising kids, or maybe not, but still somehow holding everything else together. You're expected to be constantly climbing, constantly showing up, constantly "on." And meanwhile, your body shifts in ways no one prepared you for. Your energy fluctuates, your metabolism shifts, your emotional bandwidth shrinks and expands like a rubber band being stretched to its limit and snapping back again.

This chapter isn't about adding more to your plate. It's about helping you carve out room for what *actually* matters, your energy, your health, your strength. It's about habits that work with your lifestyle, not against it. The kind that flexes when life throws curveballs but still keep you grounded. And maybe most importantly, it's about learning to make peace with your body and actually listen to what it's telling you.

Let's start with food and movement, because those are often the first things to fall apart when life gets full. I can't tell you how many clients have come to me apologizing for skipping a workout or eating takeout three nights in a row. The guilt is so baked in, like they've failed some invisible health test. But the truth is, rigid routines are rarely sustainable in this phase of life. What you need are systems that bend when you need them to, but don't break.

Preparing food does not need to mean that every meal is picture perfect. It can be as simple as having of meal anchors: a protein, a veg, and a carb, that you can mix and match all week long. One night it's salmon, roasted broccoli, and quinoa. The next, it's a stir fry with leftover chicken and rice. You don't need a different meal every single night. You just need a handful of options that keep you fed and fueled.

Same goes for workouts. Some weeks, you'll feel unstoppable. You'll crush every lift, push hard on the bike, get in your steps, maybe even throw in a yoga class for good measure. Other weeks, just getting outside for a walk feels like a win. That's normal. You're human. Your workouts should meet you where you are, not punish you for where you're not.

Syncing with your cycle can be a gamechanger. When you understand the natural ebbs and flows of your energy, you stop fighting yourself. You stop forcing intense cardio when you're already wiped. You stop feeling bad for craving carbs or needing more rest. You start working *with* your body, not against it, and that's a powerful shift.

Interior team: please rework the following worksheet so it is on its own one page (front and back)

Build Your Power Habits Plan

A flexible weekly reset for energy, strength, and sanity.

Section 1: Know Your Rhythm

- What days/times do I typically feel energized?

- When do I feel drained or overwhelmed?

- What are the top 3 stressors in my current season?

Section 2: Food Anchors

Choose your go-to proteins, veggies, and carbs for the week.

Proteins	Veggies	Carbs

Section 3: Movement Menu

Pick from this week's realistic options:

[   ] Strength workout

[   ] Long walk or hike

[   ] Stretch + mobility

[   ] Yoga or Pilates

[   ] 10-minute movement snack

[   ] Just get outside today

Build Your Power Habits Plan

A flexible weekly reset for energy, strength, and sanity.

Section 4: Micro Moments for Nervous System Reset

Which ones can I use this week?

[   ] 3 deep breaths at a red light

[   ] Silent 5 minutes on the floor

[   ] Stretch while the coffee brews

[   ] Say "'no" without a long excuse

[   ] Go outside, even just to stand in the sun

Section 5: Boundary Check-In

- Who drains me? Who lifts me up?

[   ] I will create space from...

[   ] I will intentionally spend time with...

Section 6: Body Feedback Tracker (Optional)

Energy:							
Mood:							
Body Signals:							

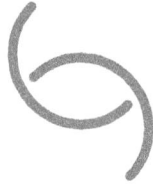

PART IV
PERIMENOPAUSE & MENOPAUSE: THE TRANSITION YEARS

CHAPTER 9
WHAT'S HAPPENING TO ME?

Melissa is 41. She's consistent with her training, eats well, manages a busy household and job, and rarely complains. But during one of our recent check-ins, she paused and said, "I think I had my first hot flash last night."

She described waking up in the middle of the night, suddenly feeling hot and flushed with damp sheets and a racing heart. It passed quickly, but she couldn't fall back asleep. She didn't have a fever. She wasn't sick. It just felt different.

Her next question was one I hear more often than you'd think: "Is this perimenopause?"

The short answer? It could be.

Most women don't expect perimenopause to start in their early 40s, or in some cases, even earlier, but that's often when the first signs appear. So many of us are caught off guard because no one really teaches us what to expect. There's no milestone or marker like there is with starting your period. Instead, it's a slow and sometimes confusing transition that unfolds over several years.

Perimenopause is the time leading up to menopause, which is officially marked by 12 months without a period. During your perimenopausal years, hormones fluctuate significantly, often more than we realize. The process doesn't look like a slow, graceful decline in hormones. Estrogen, in particular, becomes unpredictable. One month it may surge higher than usual, and the next it may crash. These highs and lows can affect everything from your energy and mood to your appetite, sleep, and how your body responds to stress. Progesterone, on the other hand, tends to decline more steadily. Since progesterone plays a big role in calming the nervous system, helping us fall and stay asleep, and supporting mood stability, its decline often shows up as increased anxiety, irritability, restless sleep, or feelings of overwhelm.

These changes can begin even when your cycle still seems regular on the surface. That's why it's easy to miss, or to chalk up the symptoms to stress, aging, or burnout.

Some of the most common early signs include:

- Trouble falling or staying asleep

- Hot flashes or night sweats

- Mood swings or a shorter fuse

More anxiety than usual

- Changes in appetite or digestion

- New sensitivities to alcohol, caffeine, or stress

- Increased bloating or breast tenderness

- Irregular cycles or heavier/lighter periods

- Brain fog or forgetfulness

None of these symptoms alone confirm perimenopause, but the pattern over time is telling. For many women, these signs show up gradually, and if you don't know what you're looking for, it can feel like you're just "losing your edge" or "not handling life as well as you used to."

To make it more confusing, many medical professionals are not trained to recognize the full scope of perimenopausal symptoms. If your bloodwork is "normal" and your period hasn't fully disappeared, you may be told everything is fine, even if you feel anything but. That gap between lived experience and clinical recognition can leave women feeling unseen, dismissed, or unsure of what to do next.

Menopause isn't a cliff, it's a transition. And while it comes with challenges, it's not the end of vitality, strength, or well-being. But it does require a new lens. The way you trained, ate, and recovered in your 20s and 30s might not work the same way now. Your body has a new hormonal baseline, and it needs different kinds of support.

We'll get into all of that in the next chapters. Before we move on, it's important to recognize that this transition is not just physical. The mental and emotional process often involves grief, identity shifts, and the need to let go of old expectations.

It's okay if this feels hard. It's also okay if it feels like a relief to finally have words for what you've been experiencing.

Perimenopause and menopause don't have to be something you simply "get through." They can be a turning point. It's a chance to rebuild your health on your own terms, with more awareness, intention, and compassion for the body you're in.

You're not falling apart. You're shifting into a new phase, and there's power to understand how to support yourself through it.

What's Happening to Me?
Self-Check & Symptom Tracker

Step 1: Self-Reflection

1. What physical changes have I noticed recently?

2. What emotional or mental shifts have stood out to me?

3. When in the month do I feel my best?

4. When do I feel the most out of balance?

5. Have I had any recent changes in:

- Period timing or flow?

- Sleep quality?

- Food cravings?

- Libido?

- Reactions to alcohol or caffeine?

What's Happening to Me?
Self-Check & Symptom Tracker

Step 2: Symptom Pattern Tracker

Sympiom	Week 1	Week 2	Week 3	Week 4
Sleep disturbances				
Hot flashes /night sweats				
Mood swings /irritability				
Anxiety				
Brain fog				
Bloating				
Breast tenderness				
Headaches				
Low energy / fatigue				
Joint or muscle aches				
Irregular cycles				
Changes in libido				

Step 3: What I Want to Ask or Learn More About

Note: Remember, this is not about diagnosing yourself. it's about learning to listen to your body and advocate for yourself, The more awareness you have, the more empowered your choices will be.

CHAPTER 10
YOUR NEW BASELINE

One of the most common things I hear from women in their 40s and 50s is: "I'm doing everything I used to do, but it's just not working anymore." And they're not wrong.

The workouts that once made you feel lean and energized now leave you drained. You're eating the same way you always have, but your body composition is shifting, especially around your middle. Recovery feels slower. Sleep is more fragile. Motivation comes and goes. You haven't changed your habits, but your results are different.

You're not doing anything wrong: your baseline has changed, and your habits may need a shift.

Menopause isn't a deficiency. It's a progression. Your body is shifting into a new hormonal landscape, and that means your approach to training, eating, and recovery shifts too. There is nothing wrong with you and you do not need to be fixed. But you do need to be supported differently.

As Dr. Stacy Sims says, *"Women are not small men."* Most mainstream fitness and nutrition advice is based on studies done on young, fit men. And for women in midlife, especially during perimenopause and beyond, those strategies often stop working, or worse, backfire. This chapter is about changing that lens. Because your body is still capable of incredible things, but the way you support it needs to evolve.

Let's start with muscle.

Estrogen plays a big role in muscle maintenance. As it declines, so does your body's ability to preserve and build muscle tissue. It's called sarcopenia, and starts as early as your mid-30s. It doesn't just affect your strength, it impacts metabolism, bone density, blood sugar balance, joint stability, and how well you age.

Strength training is non-negotiable. It's not the lightweight, high-reps "toning" routines seen in magazines. I'm talking about lifting heavy *for you*, building power, and using progressive overload to stimulate muscle growth.

Muscle is your metabolic engine. It's your bone protector. It's your confidence builder. And it sends a powerful signal to your body: *"We still need this tissue, don't let it go."*

Strength training helps to regulate blood sugar, improve sleep, and stabilize mood. It's not just physical: it's hormonal and emotional support.

Which brings us to metabolism.

It's not that your metabolism simply "slows down" with age. What really happens is a combination of muscle loss, hormonal changes, and a nervous system that's often in a state of low-grade stress. Estrogen regulates how your body stores fat and responds to insulin. As it declines, you store fat around the belly, not because you've failed a diet, but because your physiology is different.

Women refer to this as "menopause belly." And while yes, it's frustrating, it's also reversible. The solution isn't more cardio or fewer calories. It's building muscle, managing cortisol, eating enough, especially protein, and training smarter.

Women are still being told to eat less and move more. But in this phase of life, chronically under-eating and over-exercising can actually increase belly fat, not reduce it. It drives up cortisol, depletes your muscle mass, and leaves you feeling more fatigued and frustrated.

I've worked with so many women who came to me after years of cutting carbs, skipping meals, or doing high-intensity workouts every day. They felt like their body was fighting them. But once we increased their protein, introduced real resistance training, and gave their nervous system room to breathe, things shifted. Not overnight: but consistently. They felt stronger. Clearer. More themselves.

Janis started training with me in the summer of 2024. After receiving a Stage 3 chronic kidney disease (CKD3) diagnosis the year before, she completely overhauled her diet to support her health. That change led to a significant drop in body fat, but it also left her unsure of how to move forward. As a woman in her 60s, she knew she needed strength training and adequate protein, but she didn't know how to balance those needs with her condition.

At first, we used external tools. A smart scale tracked her lean mass and visceral fat. A Fitbit gave her insight into her heart rate and recovery trends. These helped her rebuild confidence and understand how her body responded to different types of training and stress.

Over time, Janis stopped relying on the numbers because she doesn't need the data anymore, she can feel it. She knows when she has the energy to train hard and when she needs to shift a tough workout to the next day. Instead of stressing over whether she is doing enough, she tunes in and adjusts with ease. She isn't just moving better; she lives with more freedom as well. She no longer feels tied to external validation or pressured to hit arbitrary goals. She trusts her body and responds in real time. That shift gave her not only physical strength but a deep sense of peace and self-assurance.

Protein

Let's talk about protein, because it's one of the most misunderstood and most important pieces of this puzzle.

As we age, our bodies become less efficient at using the protein we eat to build muscle. That means we actually need more protein than we did in our 20s and 30s, not less.

Recommended Targets:

- Approximately 1.0–1.15 grams of protein per pound of body weight per day.

- Spread out evenly across meals.

- 35 grams of protein per meal.

Not to be perfect, but to be consistent. Protein doesn't just build muscle, it supports blood sugar, keeps you full, and improves recovery. In this phase, protein is hormonal therapy.

Which leads us to recovery: the part of training that often gets overlooked, but matters just as much as the workouts themselves.

Your nervous system is more sensitive now. Sleep might be disrupted. You may feel less resilient, even if you're doing everything "right." This isn't a weakness, it's biology. And it's why recovery needs to become a priority, not an afterthought.

Recovery:

- Prioritize sleep

- Build in low-stress days

- Strength training with intention

- Fuel before and after workouts

- Let go of the guilt when your body needs to slow down

And here's where it all ties together: estrogen helped buffer the effects of stress and cortisol. It regulated your nervous system, supported serotonin and dopamine, reduced inflammation, and aided muscle recovery.

As estrogen declines, you lose that buffer. Your cortisol response can become exaggerated. Your recovery slows. Inflammation creeps in. Sleep gets lighter. And the same stress that you once brushed off now lingers in your body longer.

So many women in perimenopause and beyond feel more reactive, more tired, and less able to bounce back, even with the same habits.

To build muscle, bone density, and burn fat in this phase, your body needs a stronger stimulus: heavier weights and more protein; and a softer recovery: more rest, more nourishment, and more nervous system support.

This isn't a downgrade. If anything, it's an upgrade in awareness. It's a shift from "more is better" to "better is better." You're not starting over, you're starting smarter.

If you've been feeling stuck or like your body isn't cooperating, you need a strategy that supports the woman you are now.

You're still powerful, adaptable and worthy of care, strength, and nourishment.

Let's meet your body where it is, and build from there!

Training Smarter, Not Harder: A Sample Plan for Your New Baseline

Now that we've covered why training, recovery, and

nutrition need to shift in midlife, let's look at what that actually looks like in practice.

Below is a sample training cycle I often use with my clients. It balances the need for heavy, muscle-building strength work and metabolic conditioning, while respecting your nervous system and recovery demands—especially in the absence of estrogen.

2–3 Weeks: Progressive Training Block

These are your "push" weeks. This is where you apply the stimulus, strength, speed, and intensity, your body needs to build muscle, improve bone density, and support metabolic health.

Structure:

- **3 hard workouts within 4 days** (e.g., Mon, Tues, Thurs)

- **3 lights to moderate movement days** (mobility, active recovery, core, or low-intensity strength)

- **1 full rest day** or an easy walk/mobility combo

Key Elements to Include:

1. Strength Training (3x/week):

Heavy, compound lifts using progressive overload. Think squats, deadlifts, rows, push presses. Focus on sets of 6–12 reps with weights that challenge you.

2. HIIT (High Intensity Interval Training) (1–3x/week):

These are short bursts of hard effort followed by recovery periods (e.g., 30 sec sprint + 90 sec rest). Typically lasts 15–20 minutes total.

3. SIT (Sprint Interval Training) (1–2x/week):

More intense than HIIT. These are *all-out* efforts for 10–20 seconds with full recovery (2–4 minutes between sprints). Done 4–6 times max.

Think: bike sprints, prowler pushes, or hill sprints.

Note: *You don't need to do both HIIT and SIT every day. Choose based on energy, phase of your cycle, and overall recovery.*

Zone 2 Cardio (Daily, but not a "Workout")

Zone 2 = low-intensity cardio, walking, slow cycling, or light swimming. You should be able to breathe through your nose and talk easily.

This supports your cardiovascular health, recovery, nervous system, and metabolic flexibility. But it's not part of your high-stimulus training, it's part of your recovery baseline.

5–7 Days: Recovery Week

This isn't a "take a break and do nothing" week. It's a reload, a time to allow your body to adapt, repair tissue, and reduce nervous system stress.

In the absence of estrogen, your body is more sensitive to cortisol and slower to recover. That means adaptation takes longer, and the cost of ignoring recovery is much higher: fatigue, poor sleep, weight gain, even injury.

Your workouts during this time should feel good, not grind.

What recovery looks like:

- 2–3 light full-body strength or mobility sessions

- 1–2 short HIIT or core-focused sessions (optional, low volume)

- More Zone 2: daily walks, breathwork, restorative movement

- Mobility, foam rolling, and nervous system down-regulation

Use this week to tune in. Refer to the Protein & Strength Planning Guide and your Symptom Tracker. If your energy is high one day, do a full-body strength session. If you feel depleted, swap in a core + mobility day instead.

Recovery doesn't mean less progress, it's when the gains *happen*. Your body needs space to rebuild. Without estrogen to buffer inflammation and accelerate repair, you must be intentional about it.

Fueling for Each Phase

Progressive Weeks:

- Increase total calories, especially protein and complex carbs to support training.

- Aim for 1.0–1.15g of protein per pound of body weight per day

- Meals are well-balanced: protein + fiber + slow carbs + healthy fat.

- Pre- and post-workout nutrition are key:

  - *Before*: light carb + protein (e.g., toast + egg or banana + shake)

  - *After*: 25–30g protein + carb (e.g., chicken & rice, Greek yogurt & berries)

Recovery Week:

- Keep protein high to maintain muscle synthesis.

- Reduce carbs slightly if overall training volume drops, but don't restrict too much.

- Focus on foods that support the nervous system and lower inflammation:
  - Omega-3s, leafy greens, fermented foods, magnesium-rich options (pumpkin seeds, beans, dark chocolate).

- Hydration and electrolytes matter, especially if you're having night sweats.

Sleep Adjustments

Sleep is the foundation of your recovery: both physical and hormonal. Estrogen once protected your sleep architecture. Without it, you may wake more frequently, feel less rested, or struggle with temperature regulation.

Tips for training and sleep alignment:

- During heavy weeks, **wind down earlier** and create a sleep routine (dark room, cool temp, screen-free time).

- **Prioritize 7–9 hours**, even if broken.

- Consider magnesium glycinate, tart cherry juice, or calming herbal teas.

- On high-volume days, aim for **a short nap** or extended low-stimulus time (like reading, meditation, or walking).

Summary: Rhythm of the Month

Week	Focus	What to Expect
1–2	Build strength + intensity	Hard lifts, HIIT/SIT, challenge
3	Continue hard work or begin taper	Adjust based on energy
4	Recovery + reload	Restore, adapt, reset

Your training needs to be responsive. Honor your new physiology. Match your effort with recovery. Fuel like it matters (because it does). And remember that your body is still powerful. It just needs a smarter strategy.

CHAPTER 11
REDEFINING WELLNESS

It can be easy to mistake our hormonal shifts for a slow unraveling. You forget a word mid-sentence, snap at someone you love, lie awake at night feeling inexplicably wired, then wake up feeling heavy, like you've already used your best energy before the day has even begun. And the strangest part is that nothing in your life has really changed! Yet your body feels different, and you're not quite sure how to meet it anymore.

As a coach, I've seen this shift play out in dozens of different ways. Sometimes it's subtle, just a friend asking why her workouts leave her wiped for days. Sometimes it's bigger, a client bursting into tears, wondering out loud when she stopped feeling like herself.

I've watched that moment evolve into something else: Something bold. Something honest. Something alive. Not because everything magically gets better, but because she stops chasing who she was or 'should' be and chooses who she wants to become next.

That's what this chapter is about.

Because when the familiar cues like how you sleep, move, eat, or think, start behaving differently, it's your body whispering at you that something needs to change. A chance to redefine your wellness in a way that makes room for what's true *now*.

Wellness in this phase isn't about doing more. It's about listening more closely.

It begins, for many women, with sleep. Not the sleep you used to know, the one that carried you away for eight uninterrupted hours, but the sleep you now find yourself negotiating with. I've coached women who do everything right: no caffeine, no screens, perfectly timed magnesium, and still, they find themselves waking in the middle of the night, their minds alert while their bodies begging for rest. This isn't about poor habits or lack of discipline. It's biology. Estrogen and progesterone once worked together to regulate temperature, calm the nervous system, and guide you gently into sleep. When they decline, so does your body's ability to settle and stay asleep.

I've seen how small, consistent signals of safety can make a difference. When a woman stops fighting her sleeplessness and honors the patterns beneath it, when she builds rituals not from shame but from care, something shifts. Maybe the sleep doesn't become perfect. But the body starts to trust again. And that trust begins to ripple.

The same thing happens with stress. Most of the women I coach aren't just busy, they're carrying decades of unspoken tension in their shoulders, in their breath, in their hearts. During this transition, that tension can no longer be ignored. Estrogen once muted the volume of stress. Without it, the sound turns up. What used to feel like a manageable to do list now feels like a mountain. What used to roll off your back now sticks to your skin. Your armor is weaker, you're more exposed. Your nervous system is asking for different terms.

The old way, pushing through, muscling forward, ignoring the signs, is no longer sustainable. And deep down, you know that. I've had clients tell me they used to thrive off pressure. They wore their stress like a badge. But now? It costs too much. The edge it gave them doesn't feel sharp, it feels brittle. They start craving steadiness, clarity and softness. They ask: *What would it look like to feel regulated, not just productive?*

And slowly, they begin to find their answers. In the quiet morning walk before anyone else wakes up. In the strength session that challenges them without depleting them. In the recovery week they no longer skip, because they understand it's where the real gains happen. In the protein-packed breakfast they no longer negotiate with. In the choice to say no, not out of guilt, but out of wisdom.

These aren't hacks. They're acts of self-respect.

They're part of something bigger: a reinvention of self.

The women I work with don't just want to manage symptoms: they want to protect their long-term strength, bone health, cognitive clarity, and joy. It shifts how they view progress. Not by chasing aesthetic goals or forcing their bodies to behave like they did at thirty. But by choosing habits that feel aligned. Movements that build. Foods that nourish. Rest that restores. By asking: *Does this support who I'm becoming?*

To redefine wellness in this chapter of life doesn't mean to let go of ambition. It lets go of the rules that never worked for your physiology in the first place. It lets go of punishment-based workouts and underfed days. It moves away from goals that require constant self-betrayal.

You can still train hard. You can still build muscle. You can still enjoy food, laugh deeply, sleep well, and feel vibrant. But it doesn't come from "doing what you've always done." It honors your current biology, capacity, and needs. It comes from tuning in, honestly, bravely, consistently.

I haven't gone through menopause myself. But I've sat across from enough women to know that this isn't the end of anything. It's a reintroduction. To your strength. To your voice. To your power. And yes, to your wellness.

You do not need to be the woman you were.

You get to become the woman you are.

Let's build her with care, kindness, and love.

CHAPTER 12
A REVOLUTION ROOTED IN RHYTHM

If you've made it to this point, I want you to pause and take a breath: not just because you've finished another chapter, but because you've already begun something bigger.

You've stepped into a conversation that most women aren't invited into until it's too late. You asked new questions, not "What's wrong with me?" but "What does my body need now?" You've learned that the answers won't always come from discipline or data, but from tuning in. From noticing the subtle shifts. From rewriting the rules we've been handed.

This book isn't just about health; it's about reclaiming your relationship with your body. It's about recognizing that wellness was never meant to be a punishment, a finish line, or a race against time. It was always meant to be a rhythm. Your rhythm.

Once you stop fighting your body and listen to

it, everything begins to change. You stop chasing arbitrary goals and start anchoring yourself in intention. You stop asking how little you can eat or how much you can do, and start asking what helps you feel powerful, present, and alive.

That's the revolution. And it's already happening.

I wrote this book because I've coached enough women to see the patterns. The same confusion. The same frustration. The same deep knowing underneath it all that says, *there has to be a better way*. This is that way, not because it's perfect, but because it's yours. Built from your own cues. Aligned with your physiology. In sync with your season.

If you've felt stuck before, I hope you now feel steady.

If you've felt lost in the noise, I hope you now feel grounded in truth.

And if you've felt alone in this process, I hope you now feel held, by the stories, the strategies, and the science that finally reflects you.

What comes next?

That part is yours to decide. You might track your cycle for the first time. You might prioritize strength training or protein intake. You might walk outside every morning before the rest of the world makes demands of you. You might gather a group of women and talk openly about things you were told to hide. You might rest more. Laugh more. Say no with confidence. Say yes to joy.

You have the map.

You've met your body with curiosity. You've learned how hormones shape your energy, your sleep, your cravings, your performance. You've seen how stress affects everything, and how nervous system regulation is not fluff, but foundational. You've discovered that rest isn't the opposite of progress. It's the container for it.

And most importantly, you've remembered that your body is not something to manage. It's something to partner with.

I don't know exactly what your next chapter will hold, but I hope it won't be written from fear. It will be built on rhythm. On awareness. On care.

And I'll still be here, whether through my coaching programs, online community, podcast, or future workshops, cheering you on and offering support as you keep walking this path.

You don't have to do it all at once. Just begin again. With one step. One meal. One breath. One lift. One moment to listen.

The revolution doesn't start with what you do.

It starts with how you *tune in*.

Stop chasing someone else's version of health, and start building your own.

Rooted in rhythm. Powered by you.

AUTHOR'S NOTE

Dear Reader,

This book was a labour of love, shaped by years of coaching, learning, listening, and living in a female body. Every chapter carries pieces of my own journey, the voices of women I've worked with, and the lessons I wish someone had handed me much earlier.

I didn't just write *about* working with your body, I wrote this book *with* mine. I drafted every word during my creative, follicular phase, when my energy felt expansive and ideas flowed easily. I edited during my organized, detail-focused luteal phase, when I had the clarity to refine and reshape. I lived the rhythm I'm teaching you, page by page.

My deepest hope is that this book feels like a permission slip. To listen to your body. To take up space. To rewrite the rules. To rest without guilt and move with intention. To feed yourself well, not out of control, but out of care.

You deserve to feel strong, supported, and at home

in your body, not just in one season of life, but in all of them.

If even one page helps you feel seen, empowered, or simply understood, then every late night and long edit was worth it.

Thank you for reading. Thank you for trusting me with your time and attention. And most of all, thank you for showing up, for yourself, and for the generations of women who will benefit from the example you set.

With so much love,
Sarah

ACKNOWLEDGMENTS

Justin, thank you for always accepting me exactly as I am. You've given me support, space, and strength to grow into the woman I aspire to be, and you've never tried to dim that. You are my rock and your quiet support is the reason I had the capacity to write this. I couldn't have done it without you.

Auntie Nadine, your ability to balance your career, raise a family, maintain strong friendships and still throw the most magical, soul-filling parties has always inspired me. But more than that, thank you for editing this book with so much care and attention. You believed in this project and in me, and I cannot thank you enough.

To Lucky Book Publishing, and especially Samantha Moonsammy, you are an absolute force. You believed in me when I didn't fully believe in myself. You've talked me up in rooms I wasn't in and reminded me of my strength when I forgot. Your confidence in me has helped build *my* confidence, and I hope you know what a difference you've made.

To Chris Leblanc, who first showed me that there was another side to movement- outside of sport and competition. You were instrumental in teaching me that how our bodies feel and function, are far more important than what they look like. My personal training job became a career, and a passion, because of your guidance. Thank you for the mentorship.

To my mom, my sisters, my nieces, my friends, and the amazing women I get the honour to coach, this book exists because of you. Your stories, your honesty, your resilience, your questions and breakthroughs, you've been my inspiration at every stage. This book is one small way I hope to give back what you've poured into me.

ABOUT THE AUTHOR

I am someone who has spent most of her life moving; sometimes loving it, and sometimes hating it. I grew up a competitive swimmer and runner, but by my twenties my body was burnt out and broken down. Stepping away from sport taught me that movement isn't just about pushing harder. It's about supporting your body so it can keep showing up for you, for everything life throws your way. I rebuilt my health through strength training, mobility work, and learning how to fuel myself with real food

Now, I help women navigate every season of life; whether that's balancing busy careers, recovering from burnout, or finding strength and confidence through peri and postmenopause. My approach is rooted in curiosity, compassion, and a belief that small, consistent changes can create incredible transformations.

I'm also the creator of Balanced Nutrition for Busy People and the Balanced Energy System Training (BEST), programs designed to help you build sustainable habits, one step at a time.

Outside of the gym, you'll usually find me hanging out with my dog, Stormy, testing healthy recipes in the kitchen (and making a spectacular mess), or curled up with my latest crochet project while binge-watching Netflix.

Let's stay connected!

Instagram: @sarah_thehealthcoach

Facebook: @sarah_thehealthcoach

YouTube: @sarah_thehealthcoach

TikTok: @sarah_thehealthcoach

thank you

Thank you for reading my book!

Dear Reader,

You made it! Thank you for walking this journey with me and for giving me the space to share my story and my passion for health. I hope these pages gave you the tools to better understand your body, the confidence to take ownership of your health, and the freedom to see movement, nutrition, and recovery in a new light.

It means more than I can express that we have shared this time together. This book was written to empower women to feel strong, capable, and informed, and knowing you have been part of that dream means everything.

If I could ask a small favor: if this book inspired or encouraged you, would you leave a review on Amazon or Goodreads? Your words not only brighten my day but also help other women discover this book. You never know, your review could be the spark someone else needs to reclaim her health and confidence.

Remember, health is wealth and motion is lotion.

Keep stacking the basics, keep trusting yourself, and keep moving forward.

With Gratitude,

Sarah

104

MY GIFT TO YOU

I am so glad you're here!

As my Gift to you, get FREE Access to the Audiobook of The Habit Revolution and other bonus content by scanning the QR Code below or visiting sarahboyd.ca

www.ingramcontent.com/pod-product-compliance
Lightning Source LLC
Chambersburg PA
CBHW022102020426
42335CB00012B/796